LOW-CARB
HIGH PROTEIN

JUICES AND SMOOTHIES
FOR ENDOMORPH

Nutritional guide to right mix proteins, fats,

and low carbs to achieve optimal health and

weight loss

JANE THORNTHWAITE

Chapter 1

Introduction to Smoothies for Endomorphs

Understanding Endomorph Body Type

The endomorph body type is one of three main somatotypes, characterized by a higher tendency to store fat, a round physique, and often a struggle with weight management. Understanding the nuances of the endomorph body type is crucial for tailoring diet, exercise, and lifestyle choices that align with personal health and fitness goals. This guide provides a comprehensive overview, offering insights into the characteristics of the endomorph body type and practical strategies for achieving a balanced, healthy lifestyle.

In the realm of health and fitness, appreciating the diversity of human bodies is crucial for crafting personalized strategies that resonate with individual goals and challenges. Among these variations, the endomorph body type stands out, characterized by its unique set of features and predispositions. Recognizing and understanding this body type is more than an exercise in categorization; it's a gateway to unlocking the potential for optimized health, well-being, and personal transformation.

The journey of an endomorph in navigating the complex world of diet and exercise is distinct. With a natural inclination towards storing fat, endomorphs often face hurdles that can seem insurmountable. However, these challenges also present opportunities for growth, learning, and profound personal development. By delving into the characteristics that define the endomorph body type, individuals can discover the most effective strategies for achieving their health and fitness aspirations.

.

The Role of Low-Carb, High-Protein Diets for Endomorphs

For individuals with an endomorph body type, navigating the complex world of nutrition can often feel like a balancing act. Characterized by a propensity to gain weight easily, especially around the abdomen, endomorphs face unique challenges in managing their weight and achieving their fitness goals. In this context, the adoption of a low-carb, high-protein diet emerges not just as a dietary preference, but as a strategic approach to harnessing the body's metabolic potential.

The essence of a low-carb, high-protein diet for endomorphs lies in its ability to regulate insulin levels and encourage the body to utilize stored fat for energy, rather than relying on carbohydrates. By reducing carbohydrate intake, the body is prompted to enter a state of ketosis, a natural metabolic process where fat is burned for fuel. This shift not only aids in weight loss but also contributes to a sustained feeling of fullness, reducing the likelihood of overeating or succumbing to cravings.

Protein plays a pivotal role in this dietary strategy, serving as the cornerstone of every meal. High-protein foods contribute to muscle repair and growth, which is essential for endomorphs who often engage in strength training as part of their fitness regimen. Moreover, protein has a high thermic effect, meaning it requires more energy for digestion, absorption, and assimilation than fats or carbohydrates. This process further boosts metabolism, aiding in weight management.

The benefits of a low-carb, high-protein diet extend beyond mere weight loss. For endomorphs, this dietary approach can lead to improvements in overall health markers, including enhanced blood sugar control, reduced blood pressure, and lower triglyceride levels. It fosters a sense of vitality and well-being, empowering individuals to lead an active and healthy lifestyle.

However, it's crucial to approach this diet with a sense of balance and mindfulness. Not all carbs are created equal, and incorporating nutrient-dense, low-glycemic carbohydrates in moderation can ensure a well-rounded diet. Similarly, choosing high-quality protein sources and healthy fats is key to optimizing nutrition and avoiding potential deficiencies.

How This Guide Can Help You Achieve Your Health Goals

This guide is designed as a beacon of light, illuminating the path towards a healthier, more balanced endomorph person. By focusing on the unique needs of the endomorph body type, it offers tailored advice that goes beyond generic health tips, diving deep into how specific dietary and lifestyle changes can transform not just your body, but your overall well-being.

At the heart of this guide is the principle that knowledge is power. Armed with a deeper understanding of how your body functions, you'll be equipped to make informed decisions that align with your health objectives. Whether you're looking to shed unwanted pounds, build strength, or simply feel more energetic throughout the day, the insights provided here are your stepping stones to success.

This isn't just about temporary fixes or following the latest diet trends. It's about embarking on a sustainable journey of transformation that respects your body's natural predispositions. By embracing a low-carb, high-protein approach tailored to the endomorph physique, you'll discover how to efficiently fuel your body, boost your metabolism, and maintain a sense of satiety and satisfaction.

In essence, this guide is more than just a resource; it's a partner in your pursuit of health and wellness. Providing you with the tools and knowledge you need, empowers you to take control of your health destiny, crafting a lifestyle that's not only conducive to your physical goals but also supportive of your overall happiness and well-being.

Chapter 2

The Science of Low-Carb, High-Protein Diets

Benefits of Low-Carb Eating for Weight Management

The benefits of adopting a low-carb diet are multifaceted and can lead to significant improvements in both physical and metabolic health. One of the most immediate effects of reducing carbohydrate intake is the decrease in water retention and bloating, which can lead to a quick reduction in weight and a feeling of lightness. This initial weight loss is encouraging for many and can be a motivator to adhere to the dietary changes.

Beyond the initial weight loss, low-carb diets have been shown to promote a more sustained and effective form of fat burning. By lowering the intake of carbohydrates, the body is encouraged to use fat as its primary source of energy, leading to fat loss over time. This process, known as ketosis in very low-carb diets, can significantly aid in reducing body fat percentage, particularly in those areas where fat is more stubbornly stored.

Moreover, low-carb eating helps in regulating blood sugar levels and improving insulin sensitivity. For individuals struggling with insulin resistance, pre-diabetes, or type 2 diabetes, reducing carbohydrate intake can lead to more stable blood sugar levels throughout the day, minimizing spikes and crashes that can lead to cravings and overeating. This regulation of blood sugar is not only crucial for weight management but also for overall metabolic health, reducing the risk of developing diabetes and other metabolic disorders.

Another significant benefit of a low-carb diet is its impact on appetite control. High-protein and high-fat foods, which are staples in a low-carb diet, are more satiating than high-carb foods. This increased satiety can lead to a natural reduction in calorie intake, as individuals feel fuller for longer periods and are less likely to overeat or snack unnecessarily. This aspect of low-carb eating is particularly beneficial for those who struggle with portion control or mindless snacking, making it easier to maintain a calorie deficit and lose weight over time.

The Importance of Protein for Muscle Maintenance and Metabolism

Protein plays a pivotal role in the body, serving as a crucial nutrient for muscle maintenance, repair, and growth, as well as being a key factor in metabolic health. Its importance cannot be overstated, particularly in the context of an active lifestyle and weight management goals.

Muscle Maintenance and Growth

Muscles are dynamic tissues that require constant repair and rebuilding, processes that are heavily dependent on protein. Dietary protein supplies amino acids, the building blocks of muscle tissue, which are essential for repairing the wear and tear muscles undergo during physical activities and for building new muscle fibers. This is particularly crucial after exercise, when muscle protein synthesis is increased, and the body needs a sufficient supply of amino acids to fuel this process. Consuming adequate protein not only supports the maintenance of existing muscle mass but also aids in the development of new muscle, which is vital for anyone engaged in regular strength training or looking to improve their physique and physical performance.

Metabolic Rate and Weight Management

Muscle tissue is metabolically active, meaning it burns calories even at rest. The more muscle mass you have, the higher your resting metabolic rate (RMR) will be, which is the rate at which your body burns calories when at rest. Therefore, maintaining or increasing muscle mass through adequate protein intake can enhance your metabolism, making it easier to manage your weight or lose fat. This increased metabolic rate provided by higher muscle mass can help in creating a calorie deficit, necessary for weight loss, without the need to drastically reduce calorie intake.

Appetite Control and Satiety

Protein is also known for its role in promoting satiety, or the feeling of fullness, more so than carbohydrates or fats. This is partly due to the body's slower and more complex process of digesting proteins, which can lead to a prolonged feeling of fullness and a reduced appetite. By incorporating more protein into your diet, you can naturally reduce your calorie intake by feeling satisfied for longer periods, which is a beneficial strategy for weight management and avoiding overeating.

Optimizing Health Beyond Muscle Maintenance

Beyond its direct benefits on muscles and metabolism, protein plays a critical role in overall health. It's involved in numerous bodily functions, including the production of enzymes and hormones, immune system responses, and the maintenance of hair, skin, and nails. Ensuring adequate protein intake is essential for the body's repair processes and for maintaining good health overall.

What Endomorphs Need to Know about Decoding Macros:

For endomorphs, understanding the role of macronutrients—proteins, carbohydrates, and fats—in their diet is essential for effective weight management and overall health. it's crucial for endomorphs who typically have a slower metabolism and may store fat more easily than other body types.

Here's what endomorphs need to know to effectively manage their macronutrient intake:

Understanding Your Body's Needs

Endomorphs tend to have a higher percentage of body fat and less muscle mass. This body composition impacts how they metabolize food, necessitating a more strategic approach to dieting that emphasizes certain macronutrients over others.

The Role of Each Macronutrient

- **Proteins:** Essential for muscle repair and growth, proteins also have a high thermogenic effect, meaning they require more energy to digest, absorb, and process than other macronutrients. This makes protein crucial for boosting metabolism and maintaining muscle mass, which is vital for endomorphs who are working on improving their body composition.

- **Carbohydrates:** While carbs are the body's primary energy source, endomorphs need to be selective about the types of carbohydrates they consume. Focusing on low-glycemic carbs that are rich in fiber (such as vegetables, legumes, and whole grains) can help manage blood sugar levels and prevent insulin spikes that lead to fat storage.

- **Fats:** Healthy fats are essential for hormone regulation, including hormones involved in metabolism and satiety. Endomorphs should prioritize sources of unsaturated fats, like avocados, nuts, seeds, and olive oil, to support their health without contributing to unwanted weight gain.

Balancing Macros for Endomorphs

Endomorphs may benefit from a macronutrient distribution that's lower in carbohydrates and higher in protein and fats. This distribution can help manage insulin sensitivity, promote satiety, and support a healthy metabolism. However, the exact ratio can vary based on individual factors like activity level, goals, and personal health.

Consulting with a nutritionist or dietitian can help endomorphs find their optimal macronutrient balance.

Adjusting and Tracking

Finding the right balance of macronutrients is a dynamic process that requires monitoring and adjustments. Tracking food intake and observing how the body responds to different macronutrient ratios can be invaluable for endomorphs. This process can help identify the most effective dietary strategy for managing weight and improving body composition.

Chapter 3

Ingredients to Love and Ingredients to Avoid

What to Include in Your Smoothies Superfoods for Endomorphs

Here are some superfoods you might consider including in your smoothies:

1. **Berries (Blueberries, Strawberries, Raspberries)**: Rich in antioxidants, vitamins, and minerals, berries are also high in fiber, which helps in weight management by keeping you full longer.

2. **Leafy Greens (Spinach, Kale, Swiss Chard)**: Very low in calories but high in fiber, vitamins, and minerals. Including leafy greens in your smoothies can increase nutrient intake without adding too many calories.

3.   **Avocado**: High in healthy fats, particularly monounsaturated fat, which can help manage hunger. Avocados also provide a smooth texture to smoothies.

4.   **Chia Seeds**: Rich in omega-3 fatty acids, fiber, and protein, chia seeds can help in feeling full and satisfied.

5.   **Greek Yogurt**: High in protein and probiotics, Greek yogurt can support muscle maintenance and gut health. Opt for the low-fat or fat-free versions to keep calories in check.

6.   **Green Tea or Matcha**: Known for its metabolism-boosting properties due to the antioxidant EGCG. Adding green tea or matcha powder can provide a caffeine boost and help in fat burning.

7.   **Nuts and Nut Butter (Almonds, Walnuts, Peanut Butter)**: Good sources of healthy fats,

protein, and fiber. They can add creaminess and flavor to your smoothies but use them in moderation due to their high calorie content.

8.   **Protein Powders (Whey, Pea, Hemp)**: Adding a scoop of protein powder can help in muscle repair and growth, which is essential for boosting metabolism.

9.   **Flaxseeds**: High in omega-3 fatty acids and fiber, flaxseeds can help in feeling full and improving digestive health.

10.   **Cinnamon**: This spice can help in regulating blood sugar levels, which can reduce cravings and help with weight management.

11.   **Ginger**: Known for its anti-inflammatory properties and ability to aid digestion and reduce bloating.

Ingredients That Can Sabotage Your Goals

Here are some ingredients to use cautiously or avoid in your smoothies:

1.   **Added Sugars**: Ingredients like table sugar, honey, syrup, or any form of added sugars can significantly increase the calorie content without adding any nutritional value. They can also lead to spikes in blood sugar levels.

2.   **High-Calorie Nut Butters and Nuts**: Although nuts and nut butter are healthy in moderation, they are very calorie-dense. Adding too much can significantly increase the calorie content of your smoothie.

3.   **Full-Fat Dairy Products**: Full-fat milk, cream, or ice cream can add a lot of saturated fats and calories. Opting for low-fat or non-dairy alternatives can be a healthier choice.

4.   **Store-Bought Fruit Juices**: Many store-bought fruit juices contain added sugars and lack the fiber found in whole fruits. They can add unnecessary calories and sugar to your smoothie.

5.   **Tropical Fruits in Excess**: Fruits like mangoes, pineapples, and bananas are healthy but high in natural sugars. Consuming them in moderation is key, especially if you're watching your sugar intake.

6.   **Flavored Yogurts**: Flavored and sweetened yogurts can contain as much sugar as a dessert. Opt for plain, unsweetened varieties to avoid these hidden sugars.

7.   **Whipped Cream and Chocolate Syrups**: These are high in sugar and saturated fats.

They can transform your healthy smoothie into a high-calorie treat.

8. **Commercial Smoothie Mixes**: Some mixes can contain added sugars, artificial flavors, and preservatives. Making smoothies from scratch with whole ingredients is a healthier option.

9. **Ice Cream or Frozen Yogurt**: Including ice cream or frozen yogurt can turn your smoothie into a high-sugar, high-fat dessert.

10. **Coconut Cream**: While coconut can be healthy in moderation, coconut cream is high in saturated fats and calories.

Building Your Low-Carb, High-Protein Pantry

Building a low-carb, high-protein pantry is an excellent strategy for supporting weight management, muscle growth, and overall health, especially for those following specific dietary patterns such as ketogenic, low-carb, or high-protein diets. Here are essential categories and items to include:

Proteins

- **Lean Meats**: Chicken breast, turkey, lean cuts of beef, and pork. These are excellent sources of high-quality protein.

- **Seafood**: Tuna, salmon, shrimp, and other fish are not only high in protein but also provide healthy omega-3 fatty acids.

- **Eggs**: A versatile source of protein that can be used in numerous recipes.

- **Dairy**: Greek yogurt (low-fat or full-fat, depending on your dietary fat goals), cheese (especially hard cheeses, which are lower in carbs), and cottage cheese.

- **Plant-Based Proteins**: Tofu, tempeh, and seitan for those who are vegetarian or vegan. These can be excellent low-carb protein sources.

Healthy Fats

- **Nuts and Seeds**: Almonds, walnuts, chia seeds, flaxseeds, and pumpkin seeds are not only high in healthy fats but also contain protein.

- **Nut Butter**: Look for natural, unsweetened versions of almond butter, peanut butter, and other nut butter.

- **Oils**: Olive oil, coconut oil, and avocado oil are great for cooking and adding to salads.

- **Avocados**: High in monounsaturated fats and can be added to meals or snacks for a nutrient boost.

Low-Carb Vegetables

- **Leafy Greens**: Spinach, kale, and other leafy greens are nutrient-dense and very low in carbs.

- **Cruciferous Vegetables**: Broccoli, cauliflower, and Brussels sprouts are high in fiber and vitamins.

- **Others**: Zucchini, bell peppers, and asparagus offer variety and are versatile for cooking.

Low-Carb Fruits

- **Berries**: Strawberries, blueberries, and raspberries can be enjoyed in moderation due to their lower carb content compared to other fruits.

- **Others**: Avocado (technically a fruit) and tomatoes (also technically a fruit) are low in carbs and can be included in many recipes.

Dairy or Dairy Alternatives

- **Cheese**: Hard cheeses, cream cheese, and others that are low in carbs.

- **Milk Alternatives**: Unsweetened almond milk, coconut milk, and other nut milk that are low in carbs and sugars.

Pantry Staples

- **Low-Carb Flours**: Almond flour, coconut flour, and other nut-based flours for baking and cooking.

- **Sweeteners**: Stevia, erythritol, monk fruit sweetener, and other low-carb sweeteners for those who need a sweet taste without the carbs.

- **Canned Goods**: Canned fish (tuna, salmon), canned meats, and low-carb vegetables for quick and easy meals.

- **Protein Powders**: Whey protein isolate, pea protein, or other low-carb protein powders for shakes and smoothies.

Condiments and Spices

- **Spices and Herbs**: Most are carb-free and can add flavor to your meals without adding calories.

- **Low-Carb Sauces**: Mustard, mayonnaise (look for versions without added sugar), and others that fit within a low-carb framework.

- **Vinegar**: Apple cider vinegar, balsamic vinegar (in moderation), and other vinegar can add flavor to dishes without significant carbs.

Chapter 4

Smoothie-Making Equipment and Techniques

Choosing Your Smoothie-Making Tools

Here's a guide to selecting the essential tools for making smoothies:

1. Blender

The cornerstone of smoothie making is a good blender. Your choice will depend on your needs, budget, and the types of smoothies you plan to make.

- **High-Performance Blenders**: Brands like Vitamix, Blendtec, and high-end Ninja models are powerful enough to pulverize even the toughest ingredients into a smooth texture. They are ideal for green smoothies, nut butter, and crushing ice but come with a higher price tag.

- **Personal Blenders**: For those who make smoothies just for themselves or prefer a compact option, personal blenders like the NutriBullet or smaller Ninja models are perfect. They're easy to clean, and you can often blend directly in a cup you can drink from.

- **Conventional Blenders**: If you're not making smoothies daily or don't need to blend hard ingredients like frozen fruit or nuts, a conventional blender may suffice. They're more affordable but may not provide as smooth a texture for tough ingredients.

2. Measuring Cups and Spoons

Precision matters in recipes, especially if you're tracking nutritional intake for health or fitness goals. A set of measuring cups and spoons ensures you add the perfect amount of each ingredient.

3. Smoothie Cups or Mason Jars

Having the right container to enjoy your smoothie can enhance the experience. Insulated smoothie cups or mason jars with lids are great for enjoying your smoothie on the go and keeping it cold.

4. Reusable Straws

Investing in a set of reusable straws (stainless steel, silicone, or glass) is not only environmentally friendly but also makes drinking thicker smoothies easier and more enjoyable.

5. Citrus Juicer or Zester

If you enjoy adding a zing to your smoothies with fresh lemon lime juice, or zest, a handheld citrus juicer or zester can make the process much easier and efficient.

6. Spatula

A silicone spatula can help you scrape down the sides of the blender to ensure all ingredients are well-blended. It's also useful for transferring every last bit of your smoothie into your cup.

7. Produce Washing Tools

A colander and a vegetable brush are handy for thoroughly washing fruits and vegetables before adding them to your smoothie. This step is crucial for removing dirt and pesticides from fresh produce.

8. Nut Milk Bag or Fine Mesh Strainer

If you're into making your plant-based milk or like your smoothies extra smooth, a nut milk bag or a fine mesh strainer can remove pulp and seeds for a smoother texture.

9. Digital Scale

For those who are very precise with their nutrition or are following specific dietary guidelines, a digital scale can ensure you're adding the exact amount of each ingredient.

10. Smoothie Recipe Book or App

While not a "tool" in the traditional sense, having a collection of smoothie recipes can inspire you and help diversify your smoothie routine. There are many books and apps dedicated to smoothie recipes for all tastes and health goals.

Smoothie-Making Tips and Tricks for Busy Lifestyles

Making smoothies can be a quick and nutritious option for those with busy lifestyles, providing an excellent way to consume a variety of fruits, vegetables, and proteins. Here are some smoothie-making tips and tricks to help you streamline the process and ensure you always have a healthy option on hand, even on your busiest days:

1. Plan Ahead

- **Prep Ingredients**: Wash, chop, and freeze fruits and vegetables in advance. Freezing them not only saves time but also adds a creamy texture to your smoothies without the need for ice.

- **Portion and Store**: Portion out smoothie ingredients into individual servings and store them in freezer-safe bags or containers. Label them with the date and contents for easy selection.

2. Use the Right Equipment

- Invest in a powerful blender that can handle frozen ingredients and operate quickly to save time in the morning or whenever you're in a rush.

- Consider a blender with a smoothie cup attachment for a quick blend-and-go option.

3. Keep a Well-Stocked Pantry

- Have a variety of frozen fruits and vegetables on hand. Frozen produce is just as nutritious as fresh and can be more convenient for smoothie making.

- Stock up on your favorite protein powders, nuts, seeds, and other mix-ins to add nutritional value and flavor to your smoothies.

4. Simplify Your Recipes

- Stick to recipes with a few ingredients to save time on prep and blending. A simple smoothie can be just as nutritious and delicious as a more complex one.

- Use a base formula (1 cup fruit, 1 cup liquid, 1/2 cup yogurt or a scoop of protein powder, and a handful of greens) and adjust from there.

5. Liquid First

- When adding ingredients to your blender, start with the liquid at the bottom. This helps to prevent blade jamming and ensures a smoother blend.

6. Embrace Versatility

- Don't be afraid to substitute ingredients based on what you have. Smoothies are forgiving, and experimenting can lead to delicious discoveries.

- Use water, milk, almond milk, or coconut water as the liquid base to vary the flavor and nutritional profile.

7. Batch Blend

- If your blender is large enough, consider making multiple servings at once. You can store the extra in the fridge for up to 24 hours or freeze them for longer. Just give it a good shake or blend again before drinking.

8. Nutritional Boosts

- Add a handful of spinach or kale to any smoothie for a nutrient boost – these greens don't significantly alter the taste.

- Incorporate superfoods like chia seeds, flaxseeds, or hemp seeds for extra fiber, omega-3s, and protein.

9. Clean As You Go

- Rinse your blender and other utensils immediately after use to prevent residue from hardening, making cleanup quicker and easier.

10. Enjoy Creatively

- Change up how you enjoy smoothies: aside from drinking, you can make smoothie bowls topped with fruits, nuts, and seeds, or freeze your smoothie mixture into popsicles for a healthy, refreshing treat.

Chapter 5

Energizing Breakfast Smoothies

Green Protein Power

Ingredients:

- 1 cup spinach

- 1/2 avocado

- 1 scoop whey protein (vanilla)

- 1 cup unsweetened almond milk

- 1 tablespoon chia seeds

- Ice cubes (optional)

Instructions: Blend all ingredients until smooth. Add ice to reach the desired consistency.

Nutritional Information: Calories: 300, Protein: 25g, Fat: 15g, Carbs: 10g

Berry Almond Bliss

Ingredients:

- 1/2 cup mixed berries (blueberries, raspberries)

- 1/4 cup Greek yogurt

- 1 cup unsweetened almond milk

- 1 tablespoon almond butter

- 1 tablespoon flaxseeds

Instructions: Combine all ingredients in a blender; blend until smooth.

Nutritional Information: Calories: 280, Protein: 18g, Fat: 14g, Carbs: 20g

Tropical Turmeric Smoothie

Ingredients:

- 1/2 cup frozen mango chunks

- 1/2 banana

- 1/2 cup coconut water

- 1/4 teaspoon turmeric

- 1 scoop vanilla protein powder

- 1 tablespoon coconut oil

Instructions: Blend everything until creamy.

Nutritional Information: Calories: 310, Protein: 20g, Fat: 12g, Carbs: 25g

Cinnamon Roll Smoothie

Ingredients:

- 1 scoop casein protein powder (vanilla)

- 1 cup unsweetened almond milk

- 1/2 teaspoon cinnamon

- 1 tablespoon ground flaxseed

- 1/2 banana

Instructions: Blend until smooth and creamy.

Nutritional Information: Calories: 275, Protein: 24g, Fat: 7g, Carbs: 25g

Keto Avocado Green Tea Smoothie

Ingredients:

- 1/2 avocado
- 1 cup spinach
- 1 scoop collagen peptides
- 1 cup brewed green tea (cooled)
- Stevia (to taste)

Instructions: Blend all ingredients until smooth.

Nutritional Information: Calories: 220, Protein: 20g, Fat: 14g, Carbs: 8g

Pumpkin Spice Protein

Ingredients:

- 1/2 cup pumpkin puree

- 1 scoop vanilla protein powder

- 1 cup unsweetened almond milk

- 1/2 teaspoon pumpkin pie spice

- 1 tablespoon almond butter

Instructions: Blend until smooth and creamy.

Nutritional Information: Calories: 315, Protein: 25g, Fat: 15g, Carbs: 20g

Zesty Lemon Blueberry

Ingredients:

- 1/2 cup blueberries

- 1/4 cup Greek yogurt

- 1 cup water

- 1 scoop whey protein (vanilla)

- Zest of 1 lemon

Instructions: Blend until smooth.

Nutritional Information: Calories: 250, Protein: 22g, Fat: 2g, Carbs: 25g

Cocoa Flax Smoothie

Ingredients:

- 1 tablespoon cocoa powder
- 1 tablespoon flaxseed meal
- 1 scoop of chocolate protein powder
- 1 cup unsweetened almond milk
- Ice cubes (optional)

Instructions: Blend all ingredients until smooth.

Nutritional Information: Calories: 275, Protein: 23g, Fat: 9g, Carbs: 15g

Spicy Ginger Smoothie

Ingredients:

- 1/2 banana

- 1/2 cup Greek yogurt

- 1 teaspoon grated ginger

- 1 scoop vanilla protein powder

- 1 cup almond milk

Instructions: Blend until smooth.

Nutritional Information: Calories: 280, Protein: 25g, Fat: 3g, Carbs: 30g

Cool Cucumber Mint

Ingredients:

- 1/2 cucumber

- 1/4 cup mint leaves

- 1 scoop whey protein (vanilla)

- 1 cup unsweetened almond milk

- Stevia (to taste)

Instructions: Blend all ingredients until smooth.

Nutritional Information: Calories: 200, Protein: 22g, Fat: 5g, Carbs: 10g

Chapter 6

Hunger-Busting Snack Smoothies

. Almond Joy Protein Smoothie

Ingredients:

- 1 scoop of chocolate protein powder

- 1 cup unsweetened almond milk

- 1 tablespoon almond butter

- 1 tablespoon unsweetened shredded coconut

- Ice cubes (optional)

Instructions: Blend all ingredients until smooth.

Nutritional Information: Calories: 280, Protein: 20g, Fat: 15g, Carbs: 8g

Chia Seed Berry Smoothie

Ingredients:

- 1/2 cup mixed berries (frozen)

- 1 tablespoon chia seeds

- 1 cup spinach

- 1 cup unsweetened almond milk

- 1 scoop vanilla protein powder

Instructions: Blend until smooth.

Nutritional Information: Calories: 270, Protein: 22g, Fat: 9g, Carbs: 20g

Avocado Lime Refreshment

Ingredients:

- 1/2 avocado

- Juice of 1 lime

- 1 cup unsweetened almond milk

- 1 scoop vanilla protein powder

- Ice cubes (optional)

- Stevia (to taste)

Instructions: Blend all ingredients until creamy.

Nutritional Information: Calories: 300, Protein: 20g, Fat: 15g, Carbs: 12g

Peanut Butter Cup Smoothie

Ingredients:

- 1 scoop of chocolate protein powder

- 1 tablespoon natural peanut butter

- 1 cup unsweetened almond milk

- Ice cubes (optional)

Instructions: Blend until smooth.

Nutritional Information: Calories: 280, Protein: 23g, Fat: 14g, Carbs: 9g

Cucumber Celery Hydration Blast

Ingredients:

- 1/2 cucumber

- 2 stalks celery

- 1 scoop green superfood powder

- 1 cup water

- Ice cubes (optional)

Instructions: Blend all ingredients until smooth.

Nutritional Information: Calories: 100, Protein: 5g, Fat: 1g, Carbs: 15g

Golden Milk Turmeric Smoothie

Ingredients:

- 1 cup unsweetened almond milk

- 1/2 teaspoon turmeric

- 1/4 teaspoon cinnamon

- 1 tablespoon almond butter

- Stevia (to taste)

- 1 scoop vanilla protein powder

Instructions: Warm the almond milk slightly, then blend with the rest of the ingredients.

Nutritional Information: Calories: 250, Protein: 20g, Fat: 14g, Carbs: 8g

Mint Chocolate Chip Protein

Ingredients:

- 1 scoop of chocolate protein powder

- 1 cup spinach

- 1/4 cup mint leaves

- 1 cup unsweetened almond milk

- Ice cubes (optional)

Instructions: Blend until smooth.

Nutritional Information: Calories: 220, Protein: 21g, Fat: 7g, Carbs: 10g

Spiced Apple Pie Smoothie

Ingredients:

- 1/2 cup unsweetened applesauce

- 1/4 teaspoon cinnamon

- 1/4 teaspoon nutmeg

- 1 scoop vanilla protein powder

- 1 cup unsweetened almond milk

- Ice cubes (optional)

Instructions: Blend all ingredients until smooth.

Nutritional Information: Calories: 250, Protein: 20g, Fat: 3g, Carbs: 25g

Zesty Orange Creamsicle

Ingredients:

- Juice of 1 orange

- 1 scoop vanilla protein powder

- 1/2 cup Greek yogurt

- 1/2 teaspoon vanilla extract

- Ice cubes (optional)

Instructions: Blend all ingredients until smooth.

Nutritional Information: Calories: 280, Protein: 30g, Fat: 3g, Carbs: 25g

Beetroot and Berry Flush

Ingredients:

- 1/2 small beetroot

- 1/2 cup mixed berries

- 1 cup water

- 1 scoop vanilla protein powder

Instructions: Blend all ingredients until smooth.

Nutritional Information: Calories: 200, Protein: 20g, Fat: 1g, Carbs: 20g

Chapter 7

Recovery and Post-Workout Smoothies

Chocolate Peanut Butter Protein Smoothie

Ingredients:

- 1 scoop of chocolate protein powder

- 1 tablespoon of natural peanut butter

- 1 cup of unsweetened almond milk

- Ice cubes

- 1 tablespoon of chia seeds

Instructions: Blend all ingredients until smooth.

Nutritional Information:

- Calories: 300

- Protein: 25g

- Carbs: 15g

- Fat: 16g

Green Recovery Smoothie

Ingredients:

- 1 cup of spinach

- 1/2 avocado

- 1 scoop of vanilla protein powder

- 1 cup of coconut water

- Ice cubes

Instructions: Blend all ingredients until smooth.

Nutritional Information:

- Calories: 250

- Protein: 22g

- Carbs: 14g

- Fat: 12g

Cinnamon Roll Recovery Smoothie

Ingredients:

- 1 scoop of vanilla protein powder

- 1 cup of unsweetened almond milk

- 1 teaspoon of cinnamon

- 1 tablespoon of flaxseeds

- Ice cubes

Instructions: Blend all ingredients until smooth.

Nutritional Information:

- Calories: 260

- Protein: 24g

- Carbs: 12g

- Fat: 14g

Peachy Keen Protein Smoothie

Ingredients:

- 1 cup of frozen peaches

- 1 scoop of vanilla protein powder

- 1 cup of Greek yogurt

- Ice cubes

Instructions: Blend all ingredients until smooth.

Nutritional Information:

- Calories: 290

- Protein: 28g

- Carbs: 25g

- Fat: 8g

Blueberry Avocado Recovery Smoothie

Ingredients:

- 1 cup of blueberries

- 1/2 avocado

- 1 scoop of vanilla protein powder

- 1 cup of coconut water

- Ice cubes

Instructions: Blend all ingredients until smooth.

Nutritional Information:

- Calories: 280

- Protein: 22g

- Carbs: 24g

- Fat: 14g

Zesty Lemon Ginger Recovery Smoothie

Ingredients:

- 1 scoop of vanilla protein powder

- 1 cup of unsweetened almond milk

- 1 lemon, juiced

- 1 teaspoon of grated ginger

- Ice cubes

Instructions: Blend all ingredients until smooth.

Nutritional Information:

- Calories: 220

- Protein: 24g

- Carbs: 10g

- Fat: 10g

Chapter 8

Meal Replacement Smoothies

Keto Avocado Green Smoothie

Ingredients:

- 1/2 avocado

- 1 cup spinach

- 1 scoop vanilla protein powder (low carb)

- 2 tablespoons hemp seeds

- 1 cup unsweetened almond milk

- Ice cubes

Instructions: Blend all ingredients until smooth.

Nutritional Information:

- Calories: 350

- Protein: 25g

- Carbs: 10g (Net Carbs: 4g)

- Fat: 24g

Berry Nutty Smoothie

Ingredients:

- 1/2 cup mixed berries (raspberries, blueberries)

- 1 scoop vanilla protein powder

- 1 tablespoon almond butter

- 1 cup unsweetened almond milk

- 1 tablespoon flaxseed

- Ice cubes

Instructions: Blend all ingredients until smooth.

Nutritional Information:

- Calories: 320

- Protein: 27g

- Carbs: 15g

- Fat: 18g

Chocolate Coconut Protein Smoothie

Ingredients:

- 1 scoop of chocolate protein powder

- 1 cup spinach

- 1 tablespoon unsweetened cocoa powder

- 1/4 cup coconut flakes

- 1 cup coconut milk

- Ice cubes

Instructions: Blend all ingredients until smooth.

Nutritional Information:

- Calories: 360

- Protein: 25g

- Carbs: 12g

- Fat: 25g

Cinnamon Apple Smoothie

Ingredients:

- 1 apple, cored and sliced

- 1 scoop vanilla protein powder

- 1 cup unsweetened almond milk

- 1 tablespoon ground flaxseed

- 1/2 teaspoon cinnamon

- Ice cubes

Instructions: Blend all ingredients until smooth.

Nutritional Information:

- Calories: 310

- Protein: 25g

- Carbs: 25g

- Fat: 12g

Mocha Morning Boost

Ingredients:

- 1 scoop of chocolate protein powder

- 1 cup brewed coffee (cooled)

- 1/2 avocado

- 1 tablespoon cocoa powder

- 1 teaspoon vanilla extract

- Ice cubes

Instructions: Blend all ingredients until smooth.

Nutritional Information:

- Calories: 340

- Protein: 25g

- Carbs: 15g

- Fat: 22g

Zesty Orange Ginger Smoothie

Ingredients:

- 1 orange, peeled and seeded

- 1 scoop vanilla protein powder

- 1/2 teaspoon grated ginger

- 1 tablespoon chia seeds

- 1 cup unsweetened almond milk

- Ice cubes

Instructions: Blend all ingredients until smooth.

Nutritional Information:

- Calories: 300

- Protein: 26g

- Carbs: 24g

- Fat: 10g

Creamy Peanut Butter Banana Smoothie

Ingredients:

- 1 banana
- 1 scoop vanilla protein powder
- 1 tablespoon natural peanut butter
- 1 cup unsweetened almond milk
- 1 tablespoon ground flaxseed
- Ice cubes

Instructions: Blend all ingredients until smooth.

Nutritional Information:

- Calories: 380
- Protein: 27g
- Carbs: 30g
- Fat: 18g

Spinach Avocado Citrus Smoothie

Ingredients:

- 1 cup spinach

- 1/2 avocado

- 1 scoop vanilla protein powder

- 1/2 grapefruit, peeled

- 1 cup unsweetened almond milk

- Ice cubes

Instructions: Blend all ingredients until smooth.

Nutritional Information:

- Calories: 320

- Protein: 26g

- Carbs: 20g

- Fat: 18g

Blueberry Flax Super Smoothie

Ingredients:

- 1 cup blueberries

- 1 scoop vanilla protein powder

- 1 tablespoon ground flaxseed

- 1 cup Greek yogurt

- 1 cup unsweetened almond milk

- Ice cubes

Instructions: Blend all ingredients until smooth.

Nutritional Information:

- Calories: 350

- Protein: 30g

- Carbs: 25g

- Fat: 14g

Chapter 9

Juices for Endomorph diet

Green Metabolism Booster

Ingredients:

- 1 cup spinach

- 1/2 cucumber

- 1/4 green apple

- 1 tablespoon lemon juice

- 1-inch ginger

Instructions: Juice all ingredients and stir in the lemon juice at the end.

Nutritional Information:

- Calories: 60

- Carbs: 14g

- Sugars: 9g

- Protein: 2g

- Fat: 0g

Spicy Tomato Tango

Ingredients:

- 2 large tomatoes

- 1/2 red bell pepper

- 1/4 jalapeno (optional for spice)

- 1 carrot

- 1 tablespoon lemon juice

Instructions: Juice all ingredients, then add lemon juice.

Nutritional Information:

- Calories: 80

- Carbs: 18g

- Sugars: 12g

- Protein: 3g

- Fat: 1g

Refreshing Cucumber Mint

Ingredients:

- 1 large cucumber

- 1/4 cup fresh mint leaves

- 1 stalk celery

- 1 tablespoon lime juice

Instructions: Juice all ingredients, then add lime juice.

Nutritional Information:

- Calories: 45

- Carbs: 10g

- Sugars: 6g

- Protein: 2g

- Fat: 0g

Zesty Carrot Ginger

Ingredients:

- 3 large carrots

- 1-inch ginger

- 1/4 orange (peeled)

- 1 tablespoon lemon juice

Instructions: Juice all ingredients, then stir in lemon juice.

Nutritional Information:

- Calories: 95

- Carbs: 22g

- Sugars: 16g

- Protein: 2g

- Fat: 0.5g

Lemon-lime Green Juice

Ingredients:

- 1 cup kale

- 1/2 green apple

- 1/2 lime, peeled

- 1/2 lemon, peeled

- 1-inch ginger

Instructions: Juice all ingredients together.

Nutritional Information:

- Calories: 70

- Carbs: 16g

- Sugars: 9g

- Protein: 2g

- Fat: 0g

Celery Cleanse

Ingredients:

- 4 stalks celery

- 1/2 cucumber

- 1 tablespoon parsley

- 1 apple

Instructions: Juice all ingredients together.

Nutritional Information:

- Calories: 70

- Carbs: 17g

- Sugars: 13g

- Protein: 2g

- Fat: 0g

Turmeric Sunrise

Ingredients:

- 2 carrots

- 1/2 orange, peeled

- 1/2 inch turmeric root

- 1/4 lemon, peeled

Instructions: Juice all ingredients together.

Nutritional Information:

- Calories: 80

- Carbs: 19g

- Sugars: 14g

- Protein: 1g

- Fat: 0.5g

Cool Cucumber Aloe

Ingredients:

- 1 large cucumber

- 2 tablespoons aloe vera juice

- 1/4 lime, peeled

- 1/2 apple

Instructions: Juice cucumber, lime, and apple, then stir in aloe vera juice.

Nutritional Information:

- Calories: 65

- Carbs: 15g

- Sugars: 11g

- Protein: 1g

- Fat: 0.5g

Spicy Green Detox

Ingredients:

- 1 cup spinach

- 1/2 green apple

- 1/4 jalapeno

- 1 celery stalk

- 1 inch ginger

Instructions: Juice all ingredients together.

Nutritional Information:

- Calories: 60

- Carbs: 14g

- Sugars: 9g

- Protein: 2g

- Fat: 0.5g

Antioxidant Berry Blast

Ingredients:

- 1/2 cup blueberries

- 1/2 cup strawberries

- 1 small beetroot

- 1/4 lemon, peeled

Instructions: Juice all ingredients together.

Nutritional Information:

- Calories: 100

- Carbs: 23g

- Sugars: 17g

- Protein: 2g

- Fat: 0.5g

Kale and Kiwi Kick

Ingredients:

- 1 cup kale

- 1 kiwi, peeled

- 1/2 cucumber

- 1/4 apple

Instructions: Juice all ingredients together.

Nutritional Information:

- Calories: 80

- Carbs: 18g

- Sugars: 12g

- Protein: 3g

- Fat: 1g

Golden Apple Ginger

Ingredients:

- 2 carrots

- 1/2 apple

- 1/2 inch turmeric root

- 1-inch ginger

Instructions: Juice all ingredients together.

Nutritional Information:

- Calories: 90

- Carbs: 21g

- Sugars: 15g

- Protein: 1g

- Fat: 0.5g

Savory Tomato Sip

Ingredients:

- 3 tomatoes

- 1/4 cucumber

- 1 stalk celery

- 1 tablespoon lemon juice

- Dash of sea salt

Instructions: Juice all ingredients, then add lemon juice and sea salt.

Nutritional Information:

- Calories: 70

- Carbs: 16g

- Sugars: 11g

- Protein: 3g

- Fat: 1g

Sweet Spinach Detox

Ingredients:

- 1 cup spinach

- 1/2 cucumber

- 1/4 pear

- 1 tablespoon lemon juice

Instructions: Juice all ingredients, then stir in lemon juice.

Nutritional Information:

- Calories: 60

- Carbs: 14g

- Sugars: 10g

- Protein: 2g

- Fat: 0g

Fiery Beet Fusion

Ingredients:

- 1 small beetroot

- 1 carrot

- 1/2 inch ginger

- 1/4 lemon, peeled

Instructions: Juice all ingredients together.

Nutritional Information:

- Calories: 80

- Carbs: 18g

- Sugars: 13g

- Protein: 2g

- Fat: 0.5g

Watermelon Mint

Ingredients:

- 1 cup watermelon (seedless)

- 1/4 cup mint leaves

- 1/2 lime, peeled

Instructions: Juice all ingredients together.

Nutritional Information:

- Calories: 50

- Carbs: 12g

- Sugars: 10g

- Protein: 1g

- Fat: 0.5g

Cabbage Cleanse Juice

Ingredients:

- 1 cup red cabbage

- 1/2 apple

- 1 carrot

- 1/4 lemon, peeled

Instructions: Juice all ingredients together.

Nutritional Information:

- Calories: 70

- Carbs: 17g

- Sugars: 12g

- Protein: 2g

- Fat: 0.5g

Apple Celery Zing

Ingredients:

- 2 stalks celery

- 1/2 apple

- 1/4 cucumber

- 1 tablespoon parsley

- 1/4 lime, peeled

Instructions: Juice all ingredients together.

Nutritional Information:

- Calories: 50

- Carbs: 12g

- Sugars: 9g

- Protein: 1g

- Fat: 0.5g

Pear and Parsley Power

Ingredients:

- 1 pear

- 1 cup parsley

- 1/2 cucumber

- 1/4 lemon, peeled

Instructions: Juice all ingredients together.

Nutritional Information:

- Calories: 70

- Carbs: 17g

- Sugars: 12g

- Protein: 2g

- Fat: 0.5g

Chapter 10

Conclusion

By focusing on ingredients that are rich in proteins and healthy fats, while minimizing carbohydrate intake, endomorphs can effectively work towards achieving a more balanced metabolism, reducing fat accumulation, and improving overall body composition.

These smoothies not only serve as a convenient and quick meal solution but also as a strategic tool to support a healthy lifestyle. The incorporation of high-quality protein sources aids in muscle repair and growth, which is crucial for boosting metabolic rate. Healthy fats contribute to satiety, helping to curb cravings and prevent overeating. Meanwhile, the low carbohydrate content ensures that blood sugar levels remain stable, mitigating the risk of insulin spikes and fat storage.

Moreover, the versatility and variety of smoothies available mean that endomorphs can enjoy a diverse range of flavors and nutrients without feeling restricted or bored. This diversity is key to maintaining long-term adherence to a healthy eating plan. By experimenting with different combinations of ingredients, individuals can personalize their smoothie recipes to fit their taste preferences and nutritional needs.

In the context of profitability for businesses or individuals looking to market these smoothies, there's a clear opportunity. The growing awareness of the importance of personalized nutrition—coupled with the convenience factor of smoothies—creates a promising market niche. Offering customized smoothie options for different body types, with a focus on low-carb, high-protein recipes for endomorphs, can meet the increasing demand for health-focused, tailored nutrition solutions. Highlighting the benefits, such as weight management, muscle building, and metabolic support, can further attract consumers looking for effective dietary strategies to complement their lifestyle and fitness goals.

In summary, low-carb, high-protein smoothies represent not just a dietary choice but a lifestyle adaptation for endomorphs aiming for better health outcomes. For businesses, tapping into this market by providing specialized, nutrient-dense, and appealing smoothie options can yield significant returns. By emphasizing the health benefits and personalization of these smoothies, it's possible to cater to a wide audience seeking to enhance their dietary habits and achieve their fitness objectives in a delicious, convenient, and effective way.